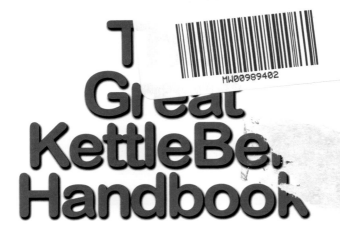

The Great KettleBell Handbook

WRITTEN BY

Jim Talo
Andre Noel Potvin

Jim Talo can be contacted with any questions at
www.humanmotion.com.

EDITED BY

EXPERT: STRENGTH TRAINING & GENERAL FITNESS
Andre Noel Potvin M.Sc., CSCS, CES

GENERAL EDITOR
Michael Jespersen
COPY EDITOR/WRITER
Keith Waddington, Kristin Warkentin

Copyright © 2008
by Productive Fitness Products Inc.

First Printing
(July 2008)

Warning:
Kettlebell training can be extremely strenuous so it is very important to first have a physician's approval. Kettlebell training can also be dangerous if the kettlebell is dropped or you experience loss of control.

Disclaimer:
The exercises and advice contained in this book may be too difficult or strenuous for some people. The authors and publishers of this book are not responsible in any way whatsoever for injuries which may occur from following the instructions herein.

Published 2008
Productive Fitness Products Inc.
18525 53rd. Avenue, Unit 120
Surrey, B.C. V3S 7A4

Productive Fitness Publishing Inc.
P.O. Box 2325
Blaine, WA 98231

E-mail: info@productivefitness.com

Visit our website: www.productivefitness.com

Info

For a listing of all the muscles used in the kettlebell exercises, visit www.productivefitness.com

TABLE OF
CONTENTS

INTRODUCTION

The kettlebell was originally used in Russia and Europe as a counter weight for agricultural scales. Being easily accessible, it gained popularity as a tool for feats of strength and competitions. In 1948, the kettlebell became the tool of choice for training elite Russian military forces. Today you can find the kettlebell in many different countries, used not only in competitions by enthusiasts, but also in sport and general fitness.

Kettlebells allow for complex full body motions that engage the major muscle groups, making it an extremely effective training device. Unlike most dumbbell exercises, muscles are forced to work as a synergistic unit across several planes of motion, all the while maintaining balance and control. Kettlebells are also one of the best tools for targeting the five components of fitness: strength, flexibility, body composition, muscular endurance and cardiovascular endurance.

A regime of kettlebell training results in an improved work capacity by building strength and endurance. The design of the kettlebell makes it particularly suited for performing foundational movements that recruit major muscle groups to work together.

In North America there is a growing awareness of the kettlebells usefulness in training for athletic performance, general fitness and everything in between. Not only are kettlebells used to improve overall performance by athletes from diverse sporting backgrounds, but also by police officers, fire-fighters and other professions requiring a superior level of physical ability.

The increasing popularity of kettlebell training for both men and women is largely due to its incredible fitness benefits and timesaving factor. Since both strength and cardiovascular systems are challenged, the result is a combined workout that saves time and burns calories. Kettlebell training is intensive, so the same work can be completed in about half the time of a traditional workout. While the kettlebell can at first seem quite intimidating, practicing and perfecting a few of the movement patterns will soon make your workouts very dynamic and fun. It won't be long before the kettlebell becomes an essential part of your fitness routine.

THE
KETTLEBELL

The shape and design of the kettlebell makes transitioning into different movements easy and fluid. Ideally, a kettlebell is a near perfect sphere with a small, flat bottom and a handle wider than one hand width.
Some things to look for in a good kettlebell include:

1. **Handle thickness.** You should be able to put your thumb over the tip of your index finger in an "Okay" hand gesture. A handle that is too thick may result in loss of grip.

2. **Handle height.** When your hand is deep into the handle, the belly of the bell should rest on the back of your forearm and not on the wrist (page 13).

3. **Distance across the handle.** To ensure smooth transitions, the gap should be neither too narrow nor too wide.

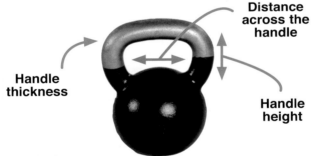

Distance across the handle

Handle thickness

Handle height

Kettlebell Styles:
Given the growing popularity of kettlebell training, manufacturers are now developing more appealing types of bells. They now come in a multitude of colors and designs.

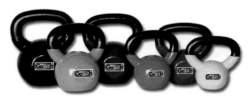

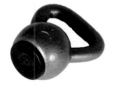

Some manufacturers have also developed soft or rubberized bottoms to protect hardwood flooring.

Competitive kettlebells are slightly more expensive than standard models and tend to retain the same spherical dimensions regardless of weight. For instance, an 18lb./8kg. bell has the same dimensions as a 26lb./12kg. bell. This consistency allows for the use of different weights without compromising technique when sports lifting or training for long duration sets. In order to maintain the tempo and duration of lifts you must acquire a certain mastery of the technique. In the context of competition, high repetitions are the supreme test of stamina and strength.

The Secret of the Kettlebell

The shape and design of a kettlebell makes transitioning from one movement to another easy and fluid. As a result, combination lifts can be performed smoothly. Kettlebells are particularly suited to movements such as "jerks," "clean and jerks" (long cycle), "clean and front squats," "snatches," and "swings" as well as "overhead presses." The same exercises would be much more difficult using dumbbells or barbells. Performing high-repetition combination exercises is a great mixture of both strength and endurance training.

Definitions relative to this book

Foundational A basic kettlebell movement upon which other kettlebell movements can be added to make a complete exercise.

Functional An exercise that replicates or closely relates to an everyday human movement in regular life or sport.

Fitness An exercise that can be performed with other weighted objects, dumbbells, etc., other than just the kettlebell.

Choosing a Kettlebell		
Strength Level	*Start With*	*Recommended Set*
Average woman	18lb./8kg.	18, 26, 35lb./8, 12, 16kg.
Strong woman	26lb./12kg.	26, 35, 44lb./12, 16, 20kg.
Average man	35lb./16kg.	35, 44, 53lb./16, 20, 24kg.
Stronger-than-average man	44lb./20kg.	44, 53, 70lb./20, 24, 32kg.
Very strong man	53lb./24kg.	53, 70, 88lb./24, 32, 40kg.

TORSO
STABALIZATION

Torso stabilization is the process of tightening the "core" muscles around your spine to protect you from injury during any lifting, pushing or pulling movements. The core muscles are grouped into two units; the inner core and the outer core (page 8). Both units need to contract in a co-ordinated manner to provide maximum protection and performance.

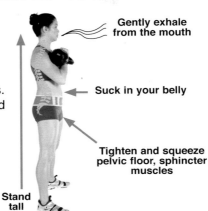

Gently exhale from the mouth

Suck in your belly

Tighten and squeeze pelvic floor, sphincter muscles

Stand tall

Why is it so important to learn this technique?

Torso stabilization is essential since the spine acts as the body's anchor from which all other muscles pull in order to effectively function. Without this muscle and spine co-ordinated effort, the risk of injury is high. Worse, our lack of fitness, combined with the degeneration processes of aging and also a poor understanding of how to tighten the core can be a recipe for disaster.

Think of the core as creating a cylinder-like squeeze around your spine. As you contract this cylinder, all sides of the muscular walls close in together to enhance the compression force and support of your spine.

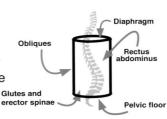

Diaphragm

Obliques

Rectus abdominus

Glutes and erector spinae

Pelvic floor

How to stabilize your torso:

Abdominals: Contract them as if preparing for a punch to the stomach.
Diaphragm: A quick inhalation through the nose to below the naval.
Spinal Muscles: Arch your lower back slightly.
Pelvic Floor: Men: imagine walking into a cold lake and squeeze.
                 Woman: stop urination mid-flow.
Glutes (buttocks): Try to lift them slightly.
Exhaling: Purse your lips and make a hissing sound.

MUSCLE
DIAGRAMS

ANTERIOR

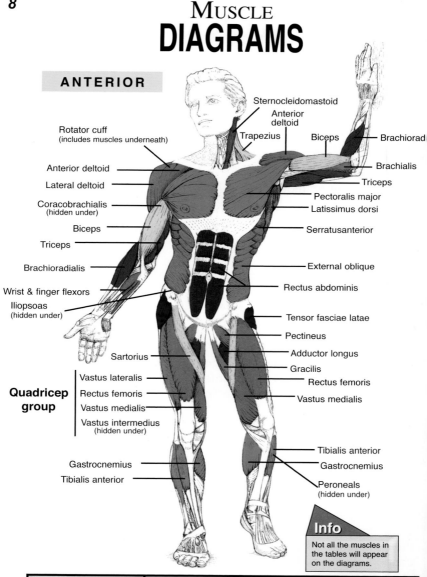

Sternocleidomastoid

Anterior deltoid

Trapezius

Biceps

Brachiorad

Rotator cuff
(includes muscles underneath)

Anterior deltoid

Lateral deltoid

Coracobrachialis
(hidden under)

Biceps

Triceps

Brachioradialis

Wrist & finger flexors

Iliopsoas
(hidden under)

Brachialis

Triceps

Pectoralis major

Latissimus dorsi

Serratusanterior

External oblique

Rectus abdominis

Tensor fasciae latae

Pectineus

Adductor longus

Sartorius

Gracilis

Rectus femoris

Vastus medialis

Quadricep group

Vastus lateralis

Rectus femoris

Vastus medialis

Vastus intermedius
(hidden under)

Tibialis anterior

Gastrocnemius

Gastrocnemius

Tibialis anterior

Peroneals
(hidden under)

Info

Not all the muscles in
the tables will appear
on the diagrams.

Neck extensors	Upper trapezius, illiocotalis cervicis, longissimus cervicis, spinalis cervicis. **Deep extensors**: semispinalis cervicis, spinalis cervicis
Neck retractors	Longus colli, Longus capitus
Scapular depressors	Latissimus dorsi, Low trapezius
Scapular retractors	Rhomboids, Mid-low trapezius
Shoulder stabilizers	Pectoralis major, Deltoid, Triceps (long head), Latissimus dorsi, Teres major, Rotator cuff
Core (outer unit)	Rectus abdominus, Erector spinae, Internal and external obliques
Core (inner unit)	Pelvic floor muscles, Diaphragm, Multifidui, Levator ani, Transversus abdominus

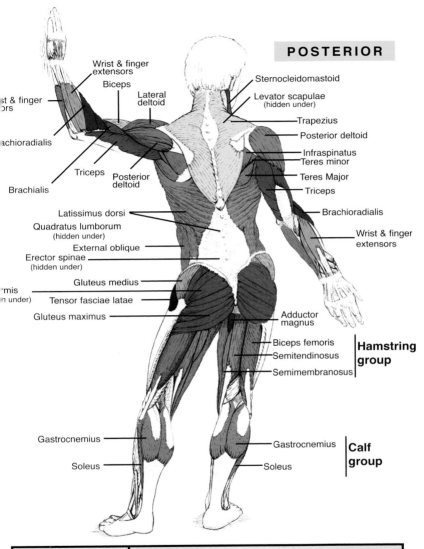

POSTERIOR

Wrist & finger extensors
Biceps
Lateral deltoid
st & finger ors
achioradialis
Triceps
Posterior deltoid
Brachialis

Sternocleidomastoid
Levator scapulae (hidden under)
Trapezius
Posterior deltoid
Infraspinatus
Teres minor
Teres Major
Triceps
Brachioradialis
Wrist & finger extensors

Latissimus dorsi
Quadratus lumborum (hidden under)
External oblique
Erector spinae (hidden under)
rmis n under)
Gluteus medius
Tensor fasciae latae
Gluteus maximus

Adductor magnus
Biceps femoris
Semitendinosus
Semimembranosus

Hamstring group

Gastrocnemius
Soleus

Gastrocnemius
Soleus

Calf group

Pelvis stabilizers	Rectus abdominus, Obliques, Quadratus lumborum, Latissimus dorsi
Spinal rotators	Obliques, Erector spinae (unilaterally), Rectus abdominus (unilaterally), Deep spinal rotators
Hip stabilizers	Hip flexors, Hip abductors, Hip extensors, Hip rotators
Hip flexors	Iliopsoas, Sartorius, Rectus femoris, Tensor facia latae
Hip adductors	Adductor brevis, Longus and magnus, Gracilis, Pectineus
Hip extensors	Gluteus maximus, Hamstrings
Hip abductors	Gluteus medius and minimus, Tensor fasciae latae, Piriformis
Ankle stabilizers	Gastrocnemius, Soleus, Tibialis posterior, Tibialis anterior, Peroneals, Extensor digitorum longus, Brevis

GENERAL

SAFETY GUIDELINES

Always warm up before you start a workout.
Try to do a total-body warm-up before you start training. A good example is light jogging for the lower body and modified push-ups (from a kneeling position) for the upper body.

Use proper posture and exercise form.
Maintaining proper posture will greatly reduce chances of injury and maximize exercise benefits. When standing, always keep your feet hip-width apart unless otherwise stated. Focus on the proper motion of the exercise. Do not sacrifice form because you want to perform more repetitions. Keep a slight arch in your back and make sure not to twist it in order to complete an exercise. It is common for many exercisers to drop and round their shoulders forward. This action exposes you to a higher risk of injury.

Breathe properly.
Never hold your breath during any part of an exercise. The rule of thumb is to exhale slowly on exertion and inhale on the return part of the exercise.

Cool down.
After completing your kettlebell workout, it is important you cool down correctly in order to prevent fainting, dizziness and muscle cramping. Perform a 5-10 minute light intensity aerobic exercise such as slow walking or biking. This activity tends to "flush-out" potentially harmful lactic acids which may still be present in your muscles.

"Set the shoulder in its socket."
This term refers to a technique you must use to ensure your upper arm (humerus) remains stable and sits tightly in your shoulder socket while performing any kettlebell exercise. Prior to performing any exercise you must set your shoulder in its socket. Here's how:

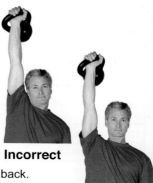

1. Lift your chest as if it is being pulled up to the ceiling by a string.

Incorrect

2. Bring your shoulders down and pull them back.
3. Hold this position throughout all shoulder and arm movements.

Correct

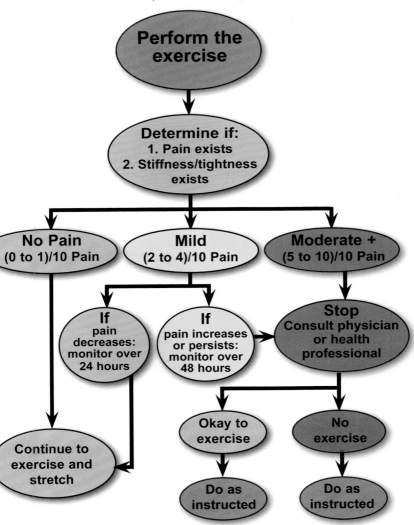

SAFE EXERCISE FLOW CHART
(Soreness Test)

Kettlebell
SAFETY

1. Common sense and good judgement must be used with all kettlebell related activities. Increase the kettlebell weight very gradually. Do not let your ego convince you otherwise.
2. If in trouble, drop the kettlebell. If you lose control of a kettlebell in mid-swing or in mid-movement, steer the kettlebell away from your body and release it.
3. Always exercise away from other people.
4. Do not use kettlebells when there are children or pets in the vicinity as they can be unpredictable.
5. Have a 15-20ft. (5-6m.) diameter of space clear of any objects.
6. Train on a surface that won't be damaged by a falling kettlebell.
7. Wear flat-soled shoes. Since many of the movements require you to transfer your weight into your heels, wearing a typical running shoe with an elevated heel may not allow you to exercise with proper form and balance.

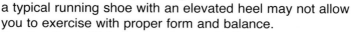
15-20 ft.   5-6 m.

8. Practice the kettlebell movements with little or no weight until you feel comfortable. Build gradually.
9. Give the kettlebell 100% of your attention. Focus on proper form and technique.
10. In order to maintain muscular control do not train to the point of fatigue.
11. Make sure you balance exercises by using both sides of the body. For instance, if you do a swing with the right hand, repeat with left.
12. Don't relax your body until you've completed the set and placed the kettlebell on the floor.
13. Keep moving after a strenuous set. Your heart rate will be racing, so keep the blood flowing by walking around.
14. When the kettlebell is overhead, keep your palm facing forward.
15. Kettlebell training requires strong core muscles for safe exercise movement. For some sample core exercises visit www.productivefitness.com.

HOW TO GRIP A
KETTLEBELL

Overhand Grip: Grasp the kettlebell near the front corner with an "Okay" gesture grip. This is a grip lock where the thumb grips over the top of the tip of your index finger. If the handle is too thick, grip the thumb over the tip of the your middle finger. Finally, wrap the remaining fingers around the handle. This is a good grip for transitioning from one move to another.

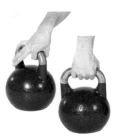

Overhand grip

Racked Position Grip: The hand sits along and deep into the handle so that the back corner and weight of the kettlebell is supported on the "heel" of the hand. Should the kettlebell handle be too wide, support the weight over the heel of the hand as best as you can.

Heel of the hand

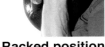

 Avoid: if the kettlebell is too high in the palm (close to the base of the fingers) your wrist will be hyper-extend. Aim to get the hand deep into the handle to set the wrist in a more neutral position.

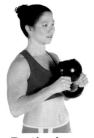

Racked position

By the "Horns" Grip: For some movements, the kettlebell may be held by the horns (where the handle attaches to the bell of the kettlebell). You may grip by the horns with the bottom either up or down.

By the horns

Palms Open Grip: When using two kettlebells, it is a good habit to keep palms open by pointing your fingers upward or subtly tucking your fingertips behind the handle. It is a painful lesson to learn should two kettlebell handles come together and a finger takes the impact.

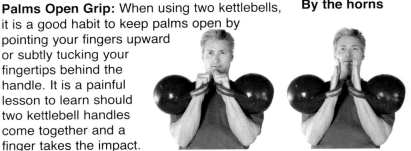

Fingers tucked   **Palms open**

How to pick up a
KETTLEBELL

Info
This is also the movement for
the deadlift exercise.

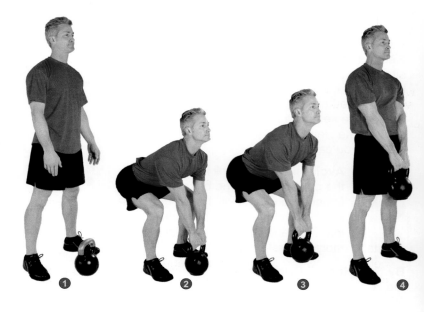

1. Start with the kettlebell placed in front and centered between
   your feet, hip-width apart ❶.
2. Keeping your shins vertical, push backward with your tailbone
   (sticking your buttocks out) while opening your chest and
   pulling your shoulders back ❷. Stabilize your torso (page 7).
3. Without looking down to find the kettlebell (feel for it), grip the
   handle with both hands.
4. Slowly return to a standing position by "pushing the floor
   away" with your heels ❸❹.
5. Reverse the motion to return the kettlebell back to the floor.

THE RACKED
POSITION

Info

This is both a holding and transitioning position.

"Nested"

Keep your wrist inside the vertical elbow line.

Women should have the majority of the weight on their sides as opposed to the chest.

Male stance   **Female stance**

Double racked position

1. After picking up the kettlebell, let the bell nest between your upper arm and forearm. Keep your wrist straight.
2. Keep your shoulder relaxed with the weight of the kettlebell settled against your side and chest. Your upper arm should be pressed against your side.

Avoid bending your wrist or letting the kettlebell hang out to the side.

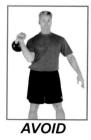

AVOID

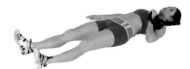

Modified Rack Position: Basically the same position as standing except you are lying down.

ASSIST TO THE

RACKED* POSITION

Info

To put the kettlebell down, perform the pick up (page 14) in reverse by sitting back into your hips and arching your back.

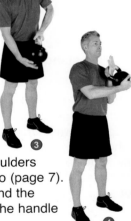

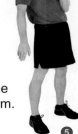

1. Start with the kettlebell placed in front and centered between your feet, hip-width apart.
2. Keeping your shins vertical, push backward with your tailbone (sticking your buttocks out), while opening your chest and pulling your shoulders back ❶. Stabilize your torso (page 7).
3. Without looking down to find the kettlebell (feel for it), grip the handle with one hand.
4. Stand up slowly, as if you are pushing the floor away with your feet ❷.
5. As you lift the bell up, lead with your thumb so the bell ends up resting on the outside of your forearm. Assist the lift with your other hand ❸ ❹.
6. Rest the weight on your chest and side while relaxing your shoulder ❺. Lightly contract your abs and gluteus muscles ("glutes"). Keep your wrist straight.

*See page 15.

LYING
PICK UP

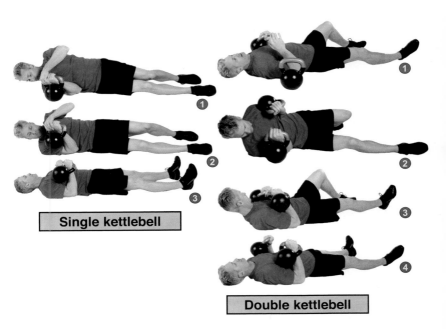

Single kettlebell

Double kettlebell

How to safely pick up a kettlebell when lying on the floor

1. Place a kettlebell on the floor and lie next to it so that it is close to your underarm when you are on your back. Stabilize your torso (page 7).
2. Roll toward the bell and grasp it with both hands❶, bringing it closer to you as you roll onto your back again❷.
3. Let the bell rest in a modified rack position❸.

When using two kettlebells

1. On your weaker side, pick up a kettlebell using the lying pick-up method (above)❶.
2. Bring the kettlebell to the modified racked position, then roll toward the other kettlebell❷.
3. Pull the kettlebell in tight to your body and roll onto your back again❸ ❹.

THE
HINGE

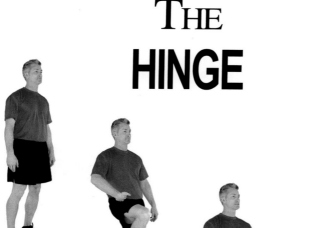

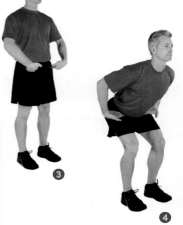

Info

The hinge is a focal point where the upper and lower body meet. It is used to maximize the power of the hip drive and engage the hamstrings, glutes, calves and muscles of the lower back, thereby minimizing the stress on your lower back.

Finding and establishing the hinge

1. Stand tall❶.
2. To find the hinge, lift one leg and place your fingers on the hip crease where your leg meets your torso❷.
3. Leaving your fingers pressed in the hinge, return to a standing position with your feet hip-width apart and toes slightly turned out.
4. Lightly press the fingers of both hands into the hip crease❸. Place most of your weight on your heels and keep your eyes looking straight ahead.
5. Keeping your shins vertical, push backward with your tailbone (sticking your buttocks out) while opening your chest and pulling your shoulders back❹.
6. Return to standing by pushing the floor away with your heels.

Hinge practice: sit back to chair

1. Stand with your back to a chair, feet hip-width apart and toes slightly turned out. Start with a light weight or kettlebell (held by the horn grip) at chest level 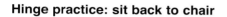.

2. Keep your shins vertical. Push backward with your tailbone while sticking your buttocks out, pushing the weight away from your chest to act as a counter balance❷. Stabilize your torso (page 7).

3. Sit back until you feel the seat of the chair under your buttocks ❸. Do not sit down. Just touch the seat, keeping your shins vertical the whole time.

4. Slowly return to a standing position by "pushing the floor away" with your heels❹.

5. When you feel more confident with this motion, increase the tempo until you are moving briskly.

KETTLEBELL
EXERCISES

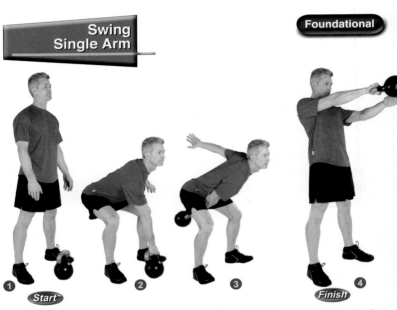

**Swing
Single Arm**

Foundational

① **Start** ② ③ ④ **Finish**

1. Pick up the kettlebell in your right hand with an overhand grip, using proper form ① ②.
2. Find a focal point somewhere in front to look at. Stabilize your torso (page 7).
3. Return to a standing position by pushing the floor away with your heels. Your arm should be straight, but able to swing freely. Let the bell sway forward as you come up. Do not lift it.
4. Sit back using the hinge motion (page 14) to swing the bell backward ③. On the return, push your heels into the floor until standing. Let your hips follow the pendulum like movement of the kettlebell. Try not to lift the kettlebell.
5. Keep your shoulder securely in the socket by not over-reaching or extending your arm forward and by keeping your shoulders square to the focal point.
6. Continue building swing momentum until the kettlebell and your arms are straight out in front of you ④. Stabilize your torso each time you reach the apex or height of your swing.
7. Repeat on the other side.

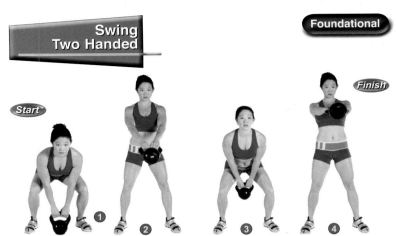

Swing Two Handed

Foundational

Start

Finish

1. Start with the kettlebell placed in front and centered between your feet, hip-width apart.
2. Lift up the kettlebell, using proper form ❶(page 14). Stabilize your torso (page 7).
3. Return to a standing position by pushing the floor away with your heels ❷. Your arms should be straight but able to swing freely. Let the bell sway forward as you straighten up.
4. Sit back using the hinge motion (page 14) to swing the bell backward ❸. On the return, push your heels into the floor until standing (see Power stance below). Let your hips follow the pendulum-like movement of the kettlebell. Do not lift the kettlebell ❹.
5. Continue until the kettlebell and your arms are straight out in front of you and parallel to the floor.

Power stance: simultaneously, drive your feet into the floor, stand tall and lift your kneecaps by contracting your quadricep muscles. Also, contract your glutes and your abs, as you exhale.

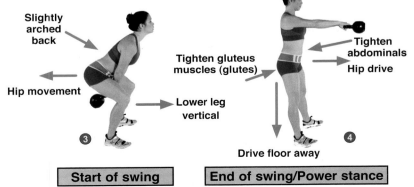

Slightly arched back

Hip movement

Tighten gluteus muscles (glutes)

Lower leg vertical

Tighten abdominals

Hip drive

Drive floor away

Start of swing

End of swing/Power stance

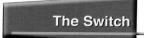

The Switch

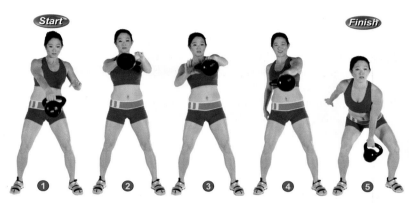

Start   Finish

1. Find a focal point somewhere in front to look at. Stabilize your torso (page 7).
2. Using proper form (page 14), pick up the kettlebell with your right hand using an overhand grip. Return to a standing position by pushing the floor away with your heels. Your arm should be straight but able to swing freely. Let the bell sway forward as you come up ❶. Do not lift it.
3. Sit back using the hinge motion (page 14) to swing the bell backward. On the return, push your heels into the floor until standing upright. Let your hips follow the pendulum-like movement of the kettlebell. Try not to lift the kettlebell.
4. Keep your shoulder securely in the socket by not over-reaching or extending your arm forward and by keeping your shoulders square to the focal point.
5. When the kettlebell reaches the apex of the swing at shoulder height, ❷ switch hands by releasing with one and grasping with the other ❸. Look directly at the handle when making the change.
6. Stabilize your torso each time you reach the apex of your swing.

Pointers

• exhale as you drive away the floor. • engage your core. • bottom of kettlebell should point at focal point at apex. • stand upright and use the power stance (page 20). • swing to chest level.

Coaching cues

• swing bell back. • drive floor away. • plank body. •
think absorb energy – redirect energy– then amplify energy.

The Clean

Info

The Clean is the most common method for getting the kettlebell into the racked position.

1. Start with the kettlebell placed in front and centered between your feet, hip-width apart.
2. Squat down and grip the kettlebell with your thumb and forefinger placed into one corner, wrapping your other fingers around as well.
3. Pick up the kettlebell and swing it back, sitting into your heels while rotating the handle so as to point your thumb toward the wall behind you ❶. Remember to open your chest as you do this.
4. Drive the floor away and tuck your elbow into your side, keeping the kettlebell close to your body as it comes up. At the same time, rotate the handle to point your thumb at the ceiling ❷. This is more of a steering movement as opposed to a pulling movement.
5. When the kettlebell reaches shoulder height (at the apex of the swing), gently catch it in the "nest" between the outside of the upper arm and forearm ❸. Bend at the knees to catch the kettlebell into this racked position. Repeat on the other side.

To steer the kettlebell back down:

1. Gently push your hips backward and let the kettlebell fall into the same pathway it took coming up.
2. As you bend at the knees, turn your thumb to point behind you as your arm straightens, letting the kettlebell swing between your legs.

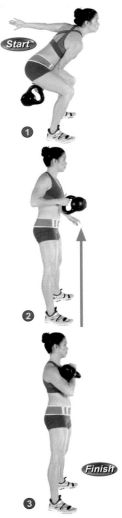

The Double Clean

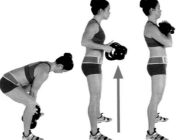

Overhead Push Press

Fitness

Info

This exercise translates into the jerk. (page 58).

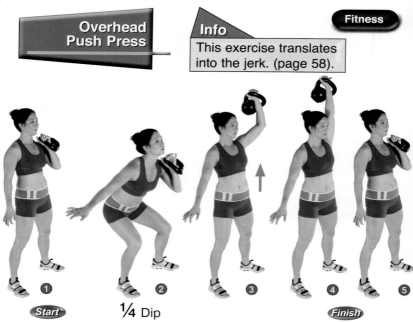

① Start ② ¼ Dip ③ ④ ⑤ Finish

1. Clean the kettlebell (page 23) to the racked position①. Stabilize your torso (page 7).
2. In one motion, dip into a ¼ squat ②and then quickly return to standing, driving your heels into the floor as you straighten your arm above your head③. Lock your elbow out when you reach a standing position④.
3. Let your shoulder settle into the joint and continue breathing.
4. Pause briefly in this upper position, then return to the racked position by bending your elbow and lowering the bell as you do a ¼ squat dip to catch the bell into the racked position⑤.
5. Keep your wrist straight in the racked position. Repeat on the other side.

Advanced

Using two kettlebells

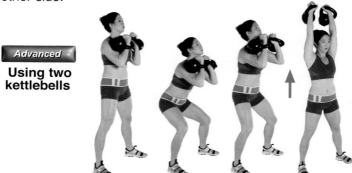

Military Press: One Arm

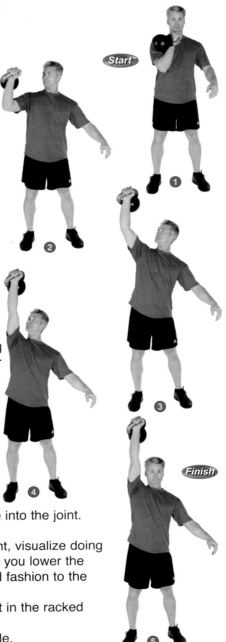

Start

1. Clean the kettlebell (page 23) to the racked position. Stabilize your torso (page 7) ❶.
2. Squeeze the handle and begin pushing the kettlebell upwards in a "C"-like movement ❷. Visualize pushing yourself away from the kettlebell and spreading the floor apart with your feet.
3. As you push up, keep your shoulder down, forearm vertical, and exhale with a hissing sound ❸.
4. Lock your elbow out once your arm is straight ❹.
5. Let your shoulder settle into the joint. Continue breathing ❺.
6. On the return movement, visualize doing a one-armed pull-up as you lower the kettlebell in a controlled fashion to the racked position.
7. Keep your wrist straight in the racked position.
8. Repeat on the other side.

Side Press

Fitness

Start

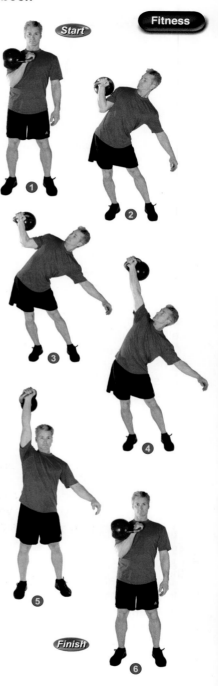

1. Stabilize your torso (page 7). In your right hand, clean the kettlebell (page 23) into the racked position❶.

2. Shift your body weight to your right leg by pushing your hip out to the right side ❷. While continuing to push your hip to the right, squeeze the handle of the kettlebell as you press it overhead. Your palm should be facing forward. Keep your eyes on the kettlebell.

3. Attempt to keep your forearm vertical as you continue pushing your hip to the side❸.

4. Extend your arm until straight and then lock out at the elbow. Lower your shoulder (page 10)❹.

5. With the kettlebell locked out overhead, stand tall❺. Ensure torso stabilization.

6. Lower the kettlebell back to the racked position❻.

7. Repeat on the other side.

Finish

Double Overhead Press

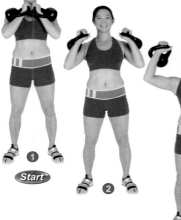
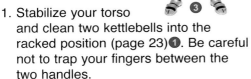
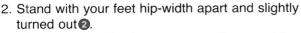

Start ❶

❷

❸

❹

❺ Finish

1. Stabilize your torso and clean two kettlebells into the racked position (page 23)❶. Be careful not to trap your fingers between the two handles.
2. Stand with your feet hip-width apart and slightly turned out❷.
3. Exhale as you slowly move your elbows out from your sides, ❸ pushing the kettlebells upwards. Squeeze the handles until both arms are straight ❹.
4. Lock out your elbows when the kettlebells are completely overhead. Lower your shoulders (page 10). Keeping your core stabilized, hold for a moment.
5. Inhale as you slowly pull the kettlebells back into the racked position❺.

Alternating Overhead Press

Fitness

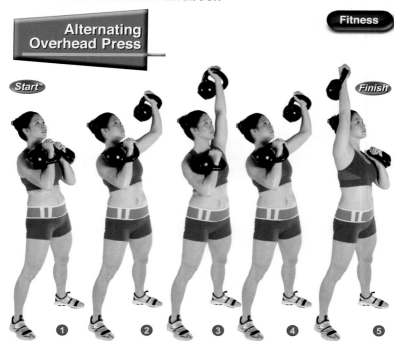

Start

Finish

1. Stabilize your torso (page 7) and clean two kettlebells (page 23) to the racked position❶. Watch that your fingers are not trapped between the two handles.
2. Begin pressing the left kettlebell overhead❷. Visualize, pushing yourself away from the ceiling as you press the bell higher.
3. Lock out your elbow when your left arm is straight❸.
4. Slowly lower the left kettlebell ❹until it returns to the racked position.
5. Pause and then repeat on the right side❺.

Variation 1

1. Press up your right side and lockout your arm overhead.
2. Press up your left side and lockout your arm overhead. (both hands are now overhead).
3. Lower your right side to racked position and then press up again, locking out your elbow.
4. Lower your left side to racked position and then press up again locking out your elbow. Repeat sequence.

Variation 2 (Seesaw Press)

1. Press up your right side and lockout your arm overhead.
2. As you press up your left side pull down on your right side at the same time. Repeat this back and forth motion.

Floor Press: Single-Arm

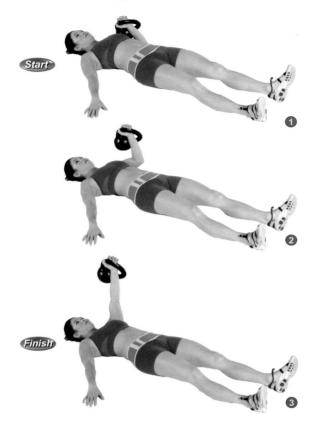

Start

2

Finish

1. Lie on the floor next to the kettlebell.
2. Use the lying pick-up method (page 17) pick up the kettlebell.
3. Once in the modified rack position, move your elbow slightly out from your side ❶.
4. Keeping your upper arm in contact with the floor, lift the kettlebell off your shoulder until your elbow is at 90° ❷. Stabilize your torso (page 7).
5. Begin the set by pressing the bell upwards until your arm is completely straight. Lock out the elbow ❸.
6. Visualize a pulling motion and slowly lower the bell back down until your elbow nearly touches the floor. Keep your forearm vertical.
7. Repeat on the other side.

Floor Press: Double-Arm

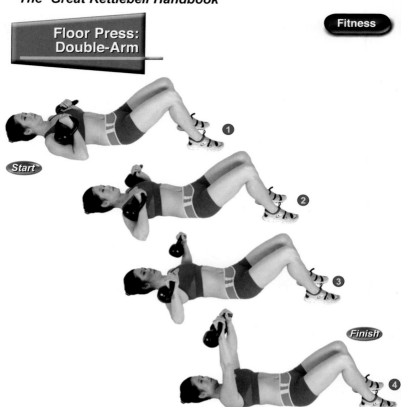

1. Place two equal sized kettlebells on the floor spaced apart so that you can lie between them.
2. Lie between the bells and use the assist method (page 17) to bring both kettlebells into the modified rack position ❶. Bend your knees and place your feet hip-width apart for stability.
3. With the kettlebells resting on your shoulders, slowly slide your elbows outwards ❷. Keeping your upper arms in contact with the floor ❸, lift the kettlebells off your shoulders until your elbows are at 90°❹. Stabilize your torso (page 7).
4. Start by slowly pressing the kettlebells upward until your arms are straight.
5. Pause briefly then slowly return to the starting position by lowering your elbows wide and out to the side. Keep the kettlebells balanced and wrists straight.
6. Stop and hold when your elbows nearly touch the floor.

Half Get-Up

Warning: use caution when holding a kettlebell overhead.

Info

Practice this exercise with no weight first before attempting it with a kettlebell.

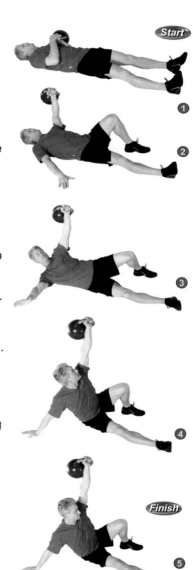

1. Lie down on the floor with a kettlebell at your left side.
2. Using the lying pick-up method (page 17), pick up the kettlebell to the modified rack position on your left side❶.
3. Bring up your left knee—on the kettlebell side—and plant your foot firmly on the floor❷. Stabilize your torso (page 7).
4. Press the kettlebell straight up and lockout your left elbow. Move your right arm straight out from your body. Keep your eyes focused on the kettlebell throughout the movement.
5. Ensure your torso is stabilized. Using your left foot, push into the floor rolling onto your side and right elbow while trying to sit up ❸.
6. Continue sitting up, supporting the weight into your right palm❹.
7. Pause in the upper position, then slowly reverse ❺ movements, keeping your kettlebell arm straight and locked out until you are lying on the floor again.
8. Repeat on the other side.

Turkish Get-Up: Lunge Style

Functional

Info

Practice this exercise with no weight first before attempting it with a kettlebell.

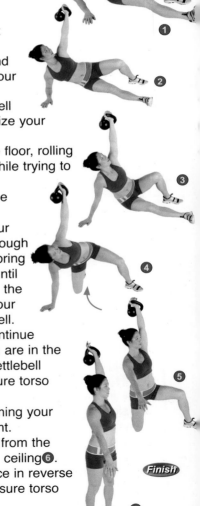

Start

1. Lie down on the floor with a kettlebell at your left side.
2. Using the lying pick-up method (page 17), place the kettlebell into the modified rack position.
3. Bring up your left knee on the kettlebell side and plant your foot firmly on the floor.
4. Press the kettlebell straight up and lockout the left elbow **1**. Move your right arm out to your side. Keep your eyes focused on the kettlebell throughout the movement. Stabilize your torso (page 7).
5. Using your left foot, push into the floor, rolling onto your side and right elbow while trying to sit up**2**.
6. Continue sitting up, supporting the weight with your right palm **3**.
7. Ensure torso stabilization. Lift your torso off the floor by pressing through your left foot. At the same time, bring your right foot under your body until you are able to put your knee on the floor so that it is directly under your hip**4**. Keep watching the kettlebell.
8. Once you have your balance, continue straightening your torso until you are in the upright lunge position with the kettlebell directly above your head**5**. Ensure torso stabilization.
9. Push up from the floor, straightening your legs until you are standing upright. Visualize pushing yourself away from the floor and reaching the bell to the ceiling**6**.
10. Stand tall. Perform the sequence in reverse and return to the beginning. Ensure torso stabilization.
8. Repeat on the other side.

Finish

Turkish Get-Up: Squat Style

Functional

Info

Practice this exercise with no weight first before attempting it with a kettlebell.

1. Lie down on the floor with a kettlebell at your left side.
2. Using the lying pick-up method (page 17), pick up the kettlebell to the modified rack position on your left side.
3. Bring up your left knee and plant your foot firmly on the floor.
4. Press the kettlebell straight up and lockout your left elbow. Move your right arm out to the side ❶. Keep your eyes on the kettlebell throughout the movement. Stabilize your torso (page 7).
5. Using your left foot, push into the floor, rolling onto your side and right elbow while trying to sit up.
6. Continue sitting up, supporting the weight with your right palm ❷. Ensure torso stabilization.
7. Lift your torso off the floor by pressing through your left foot while bringing your right foot under you and placing it on the floor, hip-width apart from your other foot ❸ ❹. Keep watching the kettlebell.
8. Using your right arm for balance, continue sitting up into a squat position until you are upright ❺. Ensure you have even balance on both feet and your torso is stable.
9. Push up from the floor, straightening your legs until you are standing upright ❻. Visualize pushing yourself away from the floor and reaching the bell to the ceiling.
10. Stand tall.
11. Place the kettlebell back on the floor.
12. Repeat on the other side.

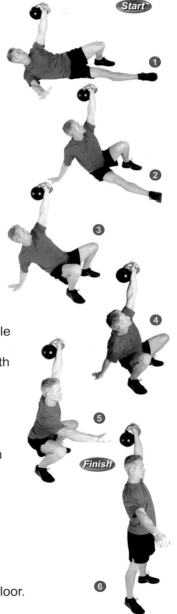

Start

Finish

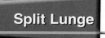

Split Lunge

Functional   Fitness

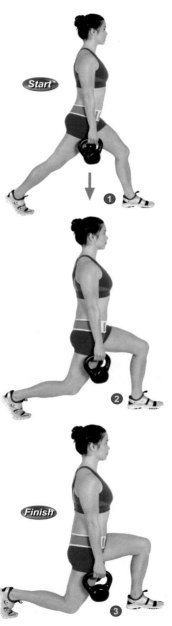

Start

Finish

Info

Watch that your pelvis remains level and does not drop or tilt to one side. Do not hold your breath and avoid poking your head/chin forward.

1. Using proper form (page 14), pick up the kettlebell with your right hand using an overhand grip. Return to a standing position by pushing the floor away with your heels❶.
2. Stand with your feet spaced about 3 feet (1 metre) apart, one in front of the other.
3. Keep your body upright and head level, chin vertical to the floor. Stabilize your torso (page 7).
4. Slowly drop your hips toward the floor until your back knee nearly touches the floor ❷ ❸. Do not let your back knee touch the floor.
5. Watch that your front knee does not go beyond your toes.
6. Pause briefly in the lower position then slowly push yourself back to the start position.

Front Squat

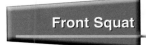

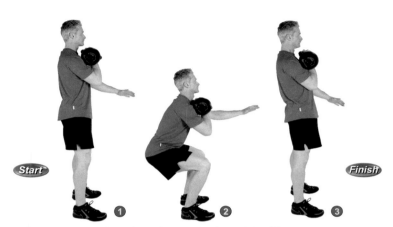

Start ❶   Finish ❸   ❷

1. Clean the kettlebell to the racked position❶.
2. Place your feet hip-width apart with toes slightly turned out. Stabilize your torso (page 7).
3. Lower yourself by pushing your hips backward, transferring the weight to your heels.
4. Open your chest and push it forward as you come down. Reach forward with your free arm to use as a counterbalance.
5. Go down as far as you comfortably can while keeping a slight arch in your back❷. Your eventual goal is to get your hip crease below the level of your knees❹.
6. Pause, then return to standing tall by pushing the floor away with your feet❸.

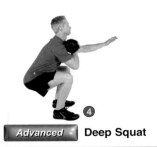

❹

Advanced **Deep Squat**

Pointers

- Lengthen your spine by thinking about moving your head away from your tailbone.
- Keep you knees in line with your toes (do not spread your knees further).

Two-Handed Variations

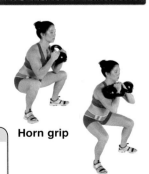

Horn grip

Two kettlebells

Overhead Squat

Functional   Fitness

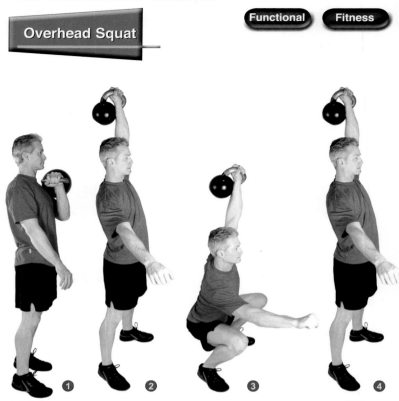

Start   Finish

1. Clean the kettlebell to the racked position (page 23). Stabilize your torso (page 7) ❶.
2. Place your feet hip-width apart with toes slightly turned out.
3. Press the kettlebell to an overhead position. Lock your elbow and lower your shoulder ❷.
4. Stabilize your torso and then lower yourself by pushing your hips backward and sticking your buttocks out ❸. Transfer the weight to your heels.
5. With your shoulders pulled back and chest open, reach forward with your free arm to use as a counterbalance.
6. Go down as far as you comfortably can. Your eventual goal is to get your hip crease below the level of your knees.
7. Pause, then return to standing tall by pushing the floor away with your feet ❹.

Face the Wall Squat

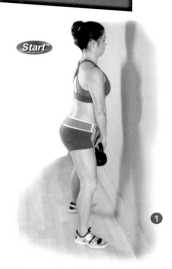

Start

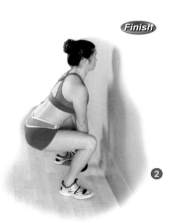

Finish

1. Place a kettlebell next to the wall.
2. Straddle the kettlebell so you are facing the wall with your toes about 3-6 inches (8-15 centimetres) away from the wall and slightly turned out. Stabilize your torso (page 7).
3. Pick up the kettlebell with both hands using an overhand grip (palms facing you) and stand up.
4. Start with the kettlebell hanging in front with your arms straight. Look down slightly ❶.
5. Squat down, pushing your knees outward (to avoid collapsing them into your arms) and arching your lower back ❷.
6. Keep you knees in line with your toes (do not spread your knees wider).
7. Pause briefly in this squat position, then return to standing.
8. Repeat this exercise without resting in the top position.

Info

Focus on sticking your buttocks out to arch your lower back.

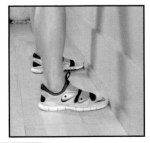

Advanced Toes touch the wall

Reverse Lunge

Fitness

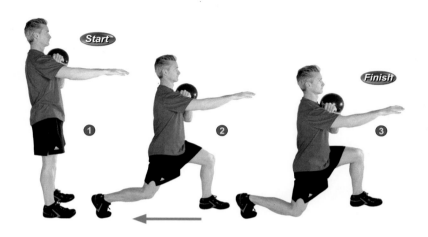

1. Clean the kettlebell to the racked position on your left side. Stabilize your torso (page 7) ❶.
2. With your right leg, step back about 3 feet (1 metre) and then lower your right knee toward the floor, stopping before it makes contact ❷. Do not allow your back knee to touch the floor.
3. In this lower position, make sure both knees are at 90° (right angles) ❸.
4. Squeeze the handle of the kettlebell and contract your glutes as you come up, pushing off the floor with your rear leg and returning to the start position.

Variation 1

Use two racked kettlebells for a more challenging exercise.

Advanced

One arm overhead

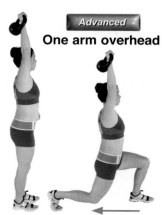

Tactical Lunge

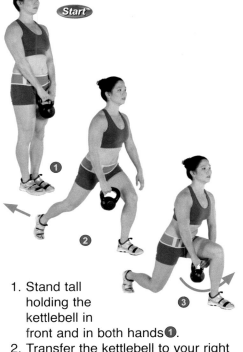

1. Stand tall holding the kettlebell in front and in both hands❶.
2. Transfer the kettlebell to your right hand as you step back about 3 feet (1 metre). Lower your right knee toward the floor, ❷ stopping before it makes contact. Stabilize your torso (page 7).
3. As you come down into the lunge, pass the kettlebell from your right hand to your left under your the left thigh❸.
4. In the lower position, make sure your front-knee is at 90° and your back knee gets close to the floor without touching it.
5. Squeeze the handle of the kettlebell and contract your glutes as you come up ❹, pushing off the floor with your rear leg and returning to the start position❺.
6. Repeat on the other side.

Romanian Deadlift

Functional   Fitness

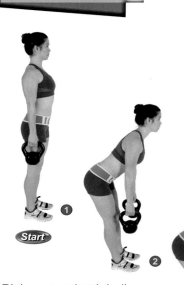

Start

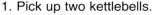

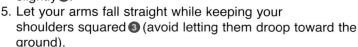

Finish

1. Pick up two kettlebells.
2. Stand with your feet hip-width apart①.
3. Stabilize your torso (page 7) and stand tall.
4. While maintaining this spinal-core stabilization, push your hips back and lower the kettlebells by bending your knees slightly②.
5. Let your arms fall straight while keeping your shoulders squared ③ (avoid letting them droop toward the ground).
6. When you reach the lower position hold the kettlebells to the side and slightly in front of your ankles④.
7. Begin the standing motion by arching your back and pushing your hips forward. Lead with your chest—sticking it up and out. Imagine pushing the floor away with your heels.
8. Keep your arms straight. Do not bend your elbows in order to lift the kettlebells.
9. Return to standing and repeat.

Suitcase Deadlift

Functional **Fitness**

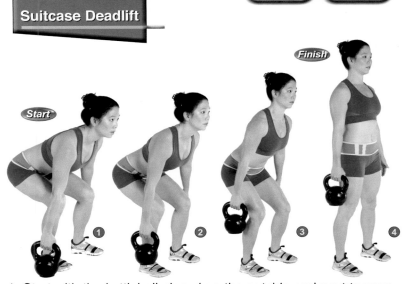

1. Start with the kettlebell placed on the outside and next to your right ankle. Stabilize your torso (page 7).
2. Squat down with your knees slightly turned out, keeping a slight arch in your back and looking straight ahead. Do not look down at the bell❶.
3. Pick up the kettlebell, keeping your shoulders squared and making sure not to lean over to one side❷.
4. Return to a standing position by driving through your heels, making a conscious effort to keep your shins vertical, hips and torso square❸.
5. Push the floor away until you return to standing❹.

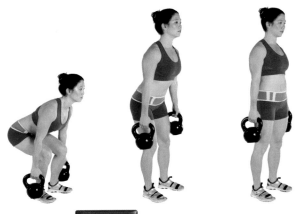

Variation **Using two kettlebells**

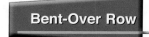

Bent-Over Row

Functional   Fitness

Info

This exercise can also be done with a single kettlebell. Use your free arm as a counter balance by reaching it forward.

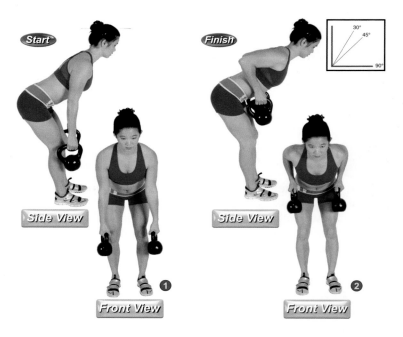

1. Start with two kettlebells placed on the outside of your ankles. Stabilize your torso (page 7).
2. With your toes slightly turned out, squat down, keeping a slight arch in your back and looking forward. Do not look down at the bells.
3. With an overhand grip, your palms facing each other, grasp the handles near the middle.
4. Maintaining a partial squat, pick up the kettlebells and raise your back to a 30° to 45° angle ❶.
5. Put your weight on your heels, making a conscious effort to keep your shins vertical, hips and torso square.
6. Lifting the kettlebells simultaneously, pull them up to the hip crease ❷.
7. Pause, then return to the hanging position and repeat.

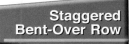

Staggered Bent-Over Row

1. Start with a kettlebell placed on the inside of your left ankle.
2. Take a big step backward with your right foot.
3. Lean forward from the hips and rest your left forearm on your left knee. Stabilize your torso (page 7).
4. With your right hand palm facing your leg, grasp the center of the kettlebell handle❶.
5. Pull the kettlebell straight up. As you lift, imagine pulling your shoulder blade down and toward the opposing buttock cheek❷.
6. Pause briefly when the kettlebell handle approaches your hip.
7. Slowly lower the kettlebell back toward the floor without setting it down❸. Continue until you have finished then switch sides.

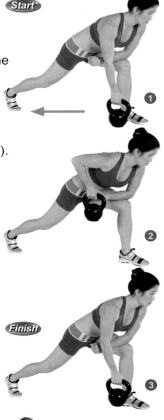

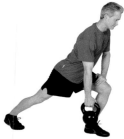

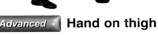 **Hand on thigh**

Planked Row

Functional   Fitness

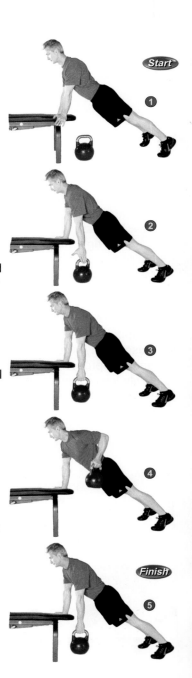

1. Start with the kettlebell placed next to a stable support, such as a bench.
2. Get into position by kneeling in front of the bench and grabbing a hold of the seat with both hands. Straighten your body until it is plank-like and rigid and using your two straight arms for support❶.
3. When you feel comfortable enough to let go with your left hand (your weight is fully supported by your right arm), grasp the center of the kettlebell handle❷. Stabilize your torso (page 7).
4. Pull the kettlebell straight up❸ As you lift, imagine pulling your left shoulder blade down and toward the opposing buttock cheek.
5. Pause briefly as the kettlebell handle approaches your hip❹.
6. Slowly, lower the kettlebell back toward the floor without setting it down❺. Continue until you finish and then switch sides.

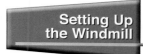

Info

Hips should go one direction. Do not twist to gain more range as this exposes the lower back to excessive loading forces.

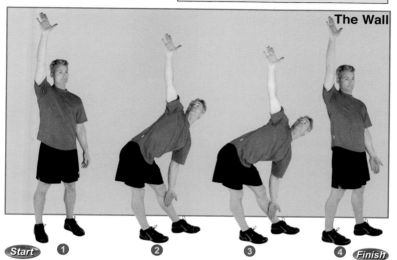

The Wall

Start ❶ ❷ ❸ ❹ Finish

Finding the "Windmill Hinge" without weight, using the wall as a guide.

1. Stand with your buttocks touching the wall. Your feet should be hip-width apart and turned slightly to the left.
2. Raise your right hand overhead, palm forward❶. Keep your eyes on your top hand.
3. Swivel your feet, using your heels as a pivot point, 45° away from your raised hand. Lift your front foot briefly so as to shift 75% of the weight to your rear foot and heel.
4. Your left buttock should now be in contact with the wall and your legs straight. Stabilize your torso (page 7).
5. Keeping your weight on your back heel, push your right hip away, allowing your left buttock to slide against the wall❷. Keep your head directly above your left foot as you slide along the wall. Note: this is a difficult motion to make, especially if you are tight in the hamstring or glutes.
6. Let your left hand keep sliding down your leg until your hips will go back no further❸.
7. Return to standing by contracting your glutes as you drive the floor away with your back heel❹.
8. Repeat on the other side.

Windmill Low Position: Option 1

Functional

1. Stand upright, feet hip-width apart, holding the kettlebell on your left side.
2. Raise your right hand overhead with your palm facing forward.
3. Swivel your feet using your heels as a pivot, 45° away from your raised hand.
4. Move the kettlebell so it is placed on the inside of your left knee with your palm facing outward ❶. Keep your eyes on your raised hand.
5. Lift your front foot briefly so as to shift 75% of the weight to your rear foot and heel.
6. Keep both arms extended without over-extending your left shoulder. Stabilize your torso (page 7).
7. Jacknife at your hips while pushing your right hip away ❷. Keep your legs straight with most of the weight on your back heel.
8. Let the weight of the kettlebell pull you a little deeper ❸. Inhale and stabilize your torso.
9. Flex your glutes and return to an upright position ❹, driving the floor away with your back heel. Stand upright ❺.
10. Repeat on the other side.

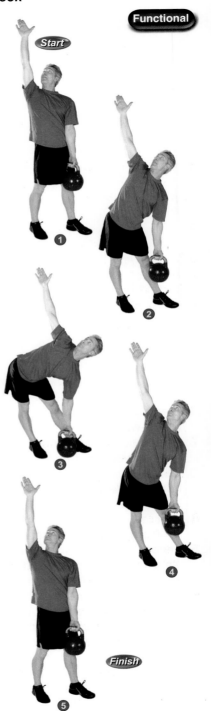

Windmill Low Position: Option 2

Start

Info

This exercise requires more mobility in the hips and hamstrings than the previous exercise.

1. Stand upright, feet hip-width apart, with the kettlebell placed next to the inside arch of your left foot.
2. Raise your right hand overhead with your palm facing forward.
3. Swivel your feet using your heels as a pivot point, 45° away from your raised hand ❶.
4. Keep your eyes on your raised hand.
5. Lift your front foot briefly so as to shift 75% of the weight to your rear foot and heel.
6. Keep both arms extended without over-extending the left shoulder. Stabilize your torso (page 7).
7. Jacknife at your hips while pushing your right hip away ❷. Keep your legs straight with most of your weight on your back heel.
8. Continue down until you are low enough to feel for the handle of the kettlebell ❸. Your eyes are still on your upper hand. Inhale and stabilize your torso.
9. Grasp the handle and lift the kettlebell to an upright position, ❹ flexing your glutes and driving the floor away with your back heel ❺.
10. Do the motion in reverse to put the kettlebell back down.
11. Repeat on the other side.

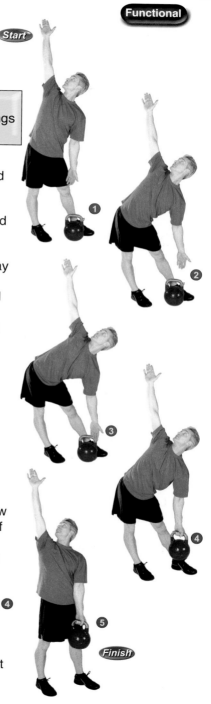

Finish

Windmill High Position: Option 1

Functional

Single kettlebell

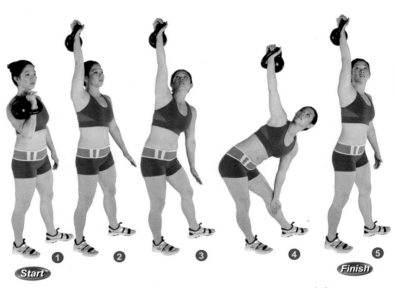

1. Start by racking the kettlebell (page 17) on your right side ①. Stabilize your torso and press the kettlebell overhead. Remember to stabilize your torso before you begin pressing the kettlebell overhead. Visualize pushing yourself away from the ceiling as you press the bell higher. Lock out your elbow when your arm is straight.
2. Swivel your feet using your heels as a pivot point, 30° to 45° away from your raised hand ②.
3. Lift your front foot briefly so as to shift 75% of the weight to your rear foot and heel.
4. Keep both arms extended without over-extending your left shoulder. Stabilize your torso (page 7).
5. Jackknife at your hips while pushing your right hip away ③. Keep your legs straight with most of your weight on your back heel.
6. Continue down, sliding your bottom hand down your inside left leg and stopping when you can go no further ④. Inhale and stabilize your torso.
7. Return to standing by driving the floor away with the back heel ⑤.
8. Repeat on the other side.

Windmill High Position: Option 2

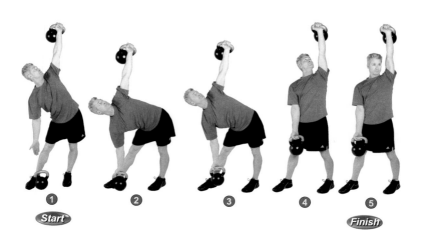

① Start ② ③ ④ ⑤ Finish

1. Start by racking the kettlebell on your left side and then pressing it overhead. Remember to stabilize your torso before you begin pressing the kettlebell overhead. Visualize pushing yourself away from the ceiling as you press the bell higher. Lock out your elbow when your arm is straight.
2. Swivel your feet, using your heels as a pivot point, 30° to 45° away from your raised hand.
3. Briefly lift your front foot so as to shift 75% of the weight to your rear foot and heel.
4. Keep both arms extended without over-extending the left shoulder❶. Stabilize your torso (page 7).
5. Jackknife at your hips while pushing your left hip away❷. Keep your legs straight with most of your weight on your back heel.
6. Continue down, sliding your bottom hand down the inside right leg until you are low enough to feel for the handle of the kettlebell❸. Your eyes are still on your upper hand. Inhale and stabilize your torso.
7. Grasp the handle and raise the kettlebell❹, flexing your glutes and returning to an upright position and driving the floor away with your back heel❺.
8. Repeat on the other side.

Setting Up the Snatch

Info

The snatch is an extension of the swing and comprised of three steps:
1. Swing   } Setting Up
2. High pull   } the Snatch
3. Clean and press out

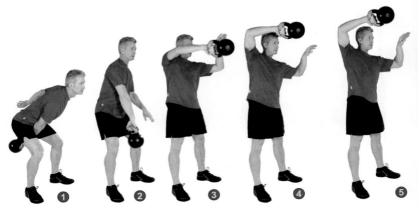

1. Stabilize your torso (page 7). Begin swinging the kettlebell using the hinge technique ❶❷.
2. Perform a few loose swings then—keeping the bell close to your body—do a high pull swing❸, driving the floor away with your heels and steering the bell up and along your body with a whip-like arm movement. If possible, keep the elbow just slightly higher than the kettlebell.
3. As the kettlebell comes up, it reaches the apex and you feel the handle push into your palm❹. Gently push the handle back and steer the kettlebell back down between your legs.
4. Continue doing this high swing, bringing the bell level with your forehead and the handle about 15 inches (40 centimetres) away from your forehead ❺.
5. Repeat on the other side.

Practice this:
1. Do a swing❸.
2. Do a high swing❺.
3. Alternate between these two movements for 10 repetitions with each arm.
4. Continue practicing these movements until it is fluid and you have mastered the motion.

Note: Practice this movement until you are comfortable and in control before proceeding to the snatch exercise (page 51).

Snatch

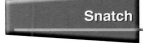

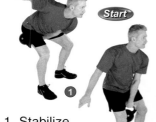

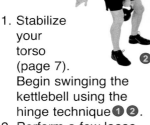

Start

Punch through

Finish

1. Stabilize your torso (page 7). Begin swinging the kettlebell using the hinge technique ❶ ❷.
2. Perform a few loose swings then do a high pull swing, ❸ driving the floor away with your heels and steering the bell up and along your body with a whip-like arm movement.
3. As the kettlebell comes up, it reaches an apex without further upward momentum and stalls in mid-air before falling again. Once the kettlebell stalls just above forehead level, punch your hand upward and forward ❹ so that the belly of the kettlebell rolls onto the back of your forearm. Do not over-tighten your grip on the handle. Allow it to move freely in your closed hand.
4. Focus on the heel of your hand doing a quick overhead press right after you punch through. This will help control the energy of the kettlebell and protect your forearm.
5. Once your arm is straight up, lock your elbow and settle the shoulder into your socket by lowering your shoulder ❺ (see shoulder safety, page 10).
6. Lower the kettlebell back to the racked position ❻ (to perform the very advanced drop-out move, see step 8).
7. Work up to performing a series of these snatches back-to-back, bringing the kettlebell to racked position and then into a swing to repeat the motion over again.
8. Repeat on the other side.

Snatch-Dropout

Foundational

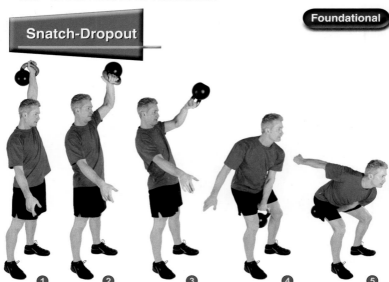

① ② ③ ④ ⑤

This progression should only to be done when you are comfortable with and have mastered the snatch on the previous page.

1. When you are in the overhead lockout position❶, gently begin to push back into your hips and let the kettlebell slowly roll off of your wrist, toward the outside of your hand (little finger side)❷, as gravity pulls it down.

2. As the kettlebell begins to fall, bend your elbow, steering the kettlebell down in front and away from your body and head❸. There should be a distance of about 18 inches (46 centimetres) between the kettlebell and your chest as it comes down.

3. As the bell descends, rotate it inward between your legs❹, hooking your fingers around the handle (DO NOT OVERGRIP) and letting it swing between your legs❺.

4. The secret is to absorb the impact by dropping back into the swing. Do not slow the kettlebell by resisting the fall with your arm or elbow movement. You should be catching the fall in your hip and bent legs. Use a gentle swing between your legs to dissipate the energy of the dropping kettlebell.

5. Use this same swing to set up the next swing and snatch.

6. When you become comfortable with the drop phase of the snatch, try doing consecutive repetitions.

7. Eventually work up to performing 30 repetitions before switching to the other side.

Single Leg Pick Up

Functional

Start **Finish**

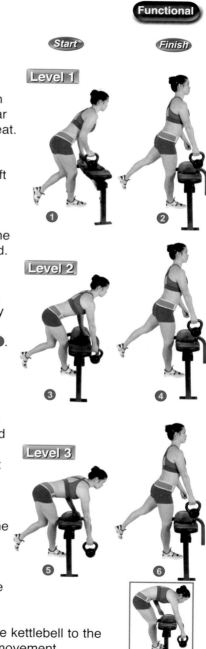

Level 1

1. Place a kettlebell on a bench with the handle perpendicular to the length of the bench seat.
2. Stand facing the side of the bench. Place your right foot under the bench and your left foot behind you (resting on your toes only).
3. Place your left hand on the bench for support and grip the kettlebell with your right hand. Your right thumb should be facing away from you.

Level 2

4. Stabilize your torso (page 7), then bend your knees slightly and hinge forward from the hips (page 18) to about 45° ❶. (Level 1=45°), (Level 2=60°), ❸ (Level 3=90°) ❺

5. Begin the lifting motion by arching your back, sticking your buttocks out and pushing your hips forward. Lead with your chest, lifting it up and out.

Level 3

6. Straighten your back leg out as you lift your toes off the floor ❷❹❻ . This engages the muscles of the back and hip extensors.
7. Keep your arms straight. Do not bend your elbow to lift the kettlebell.
8. Without resting the kettlebell on the bench, slowly lower the kettlebell to the bench again and repeat the movement.
9. Repeat on the other side.

Avoid

Fitness

Figure 8's

1. With a kettlebell in your left hand, take a wider than hip-width stance. Your toes should be turned out to the 10 and 2 o'clock positions. Stabilize your torso (page 7).
2. Sit back into your hips as if doing a squat, with most of your weight on the heels ❶.
3. Focus on a distant point and open your chest by pulling your shoulders back.
4. Begin moving the kettlebell between your legs and to the back of your right calf where you transfer the kettlebell to your right hand ❷.
5. After changing hands, begin standing as you bring the kettlebell back toward the front of your right thigh ❸. As the kettlebell moves past the front of your right knee, ❹ squat back down again pulling the kettlebell back through your legs and transferring it to your left hand ❺.
6. Continue in this manner.

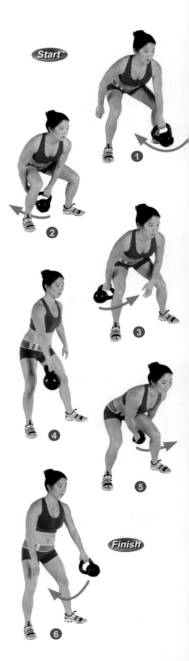

Start

❶

❷

❸

❹

❺

Finish

❻

Coaching cues
- Elbows straight.
- Do not hunch.
- Sit back into hips.
- Open chest.

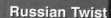

Russian Twist

1. Sit on the floor with a kettlebell between your legs.
2. Stabilize your torso (page 7). Grasp the kettlebell by the horns and bring it up to your mid-section.
3. Start by getting into a semi sit-up position, as if you were doing a sit-up and stopped just over half way. Hold the kettlebell just above your navel❶.
4. Your knees should be bent to about 90° and your feet lifted about 2 inches (5 centimetres) off the floor. Your back should have a slight arch and your chest should be broad and open.
5. In a slow and controlled movement, twist your torso to the right,❷ moving the kettlebell toward your right hip. Follow the kettlebell with your head and torso.
6. Pause briefly then return to center without letting your feet touch the floor ❸.
7. Pause briefly again and then repeat on the left side. Keep your elbows tucked into your sides❹.

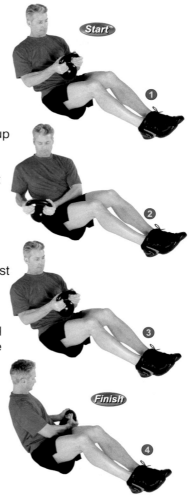

Easy Version
Keep your heels on the floor.

Difficult Version

Put the kettlebell down on the floor next to your hip, pick it up and continue to the other side and put it down again. Ensure your torso is stabilized each time.

Functional **Fitness**

Twisting Crunch

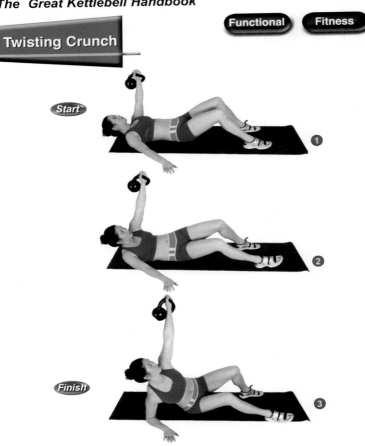

Start

Finish

1. Lie face-up on a mat with your knees bent and feet hip-width apart for stability.
2. Using the lying pick-up method (page 17) bring the kettlebell into the modified rack position on your left side.
3. Move your right arm straight out on the floor for support. Stabilize your torso (page 7).
4. Press the kettlebell up until your left arm is straight and locked out ❶.
5. Crunch up, bringing your left shoulder off the floor ❷. This motion should be initiated by your abdominals.
6. Keeping your eyes on the kettlebell, prop up onto your right arm ❸. Do not poke your chin forward as you come up.
7. Pause briefly in this position, then slowly return to the floor without resting. Keep your abdominals working. Continue breathing throughout the motion.
8. Repeat on the other side.

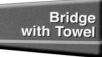

Bridge with Towel

Functional   Fitness

Info
Watch that your pelvis remains level and does not drop or tilt to one side.

Make sure to use a towel on the pelvic region

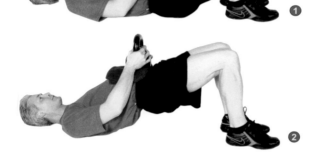

1. Lie face-up on the floor with your knees bent.
2. Place a thick folded towel on your abdomen (used to disburse the weight of the kettlebell).
3. Gently place the kettlebell on the towel, holding the kettlebell by the horns ❶.
4. Raise both hips off the floor until your knees are at 90° and your torso is perfectly straight ❷. Stabilize your torso (page 7).
5. Pause briefly in this top position, then lower back to the starting point. Continue without resting on the floor between repetitions.

Warning: use a towel or other platform on your abdomen to disburse the weight of the kettlebell.

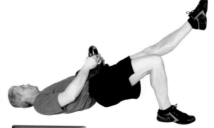

Advanced **One leg raised**

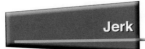

Jerk

This exercise is done in several phases resulting in one continuous movement upward, then a soft motion back to the racked position.

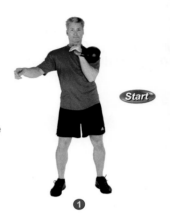

Start

1. Clean the kettlebell to the racked position❶. Stabilize your torso (page 7).

2. The four phases are:

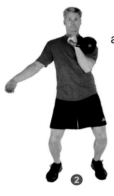

a. 1st Dip. Drop to a ¼ squat❷.

b. Then propel yourself upwards. The kettlebell begins to float out of the racked position. Your arm is loose but your hand remains on the kettlebell ❸.

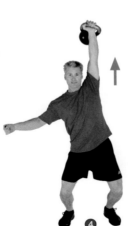

c. 2nd Dip. Let the momentum of the kettlebell continue to carry it higher as you drop back to a ¼ squat, extending your arm❹. Visualize yourself jumping down onto the floor as the kettlebell goes upward. As your arm straightens, tighten your grip on the kettlebell as you lock out your arm above your head.

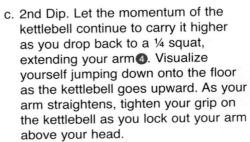

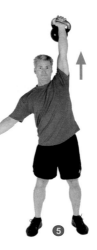

d. Return to a standing upright position with the kettlebell overhead 5. Pause.

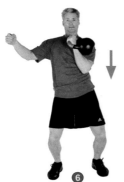

3. To return the kettlebell back to the racked position, look up slightly as you unlock your elbow letting the bell fall back into the racked position and controlling the bell as it comes down 6. As it reaches your body, absorb the impact by bending your knees.

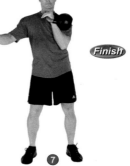

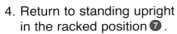

4. Return to standing upright in the racked position 7.

Info

If you have difficulty with this exercise, continue with the "push press" (page 24) as it is the precursor to the jerk.

WORKING OUT WITH
KETTLEBELLS

We strongly suggest you become familiar with all the foundational movements before attempting any of the following routines. Good technique is of the utmost importance. Only introduce new exercises into your routine when you have mastered the technique.

When using kettlebells there are two main ways to train:
1. Time based (you work until the set time has elapsed).
2. Set number of repetitions (you work until the set number of repetitions have been completed).

Traditional kettlebell training is primarily about performing a series of specific movements over a set period of time. With a fitness focus though, a set number of repetitions (reps) are performed. When you are able to successfully complete a routine, look at increasing the number of repetitions or length of time before moving to a heavier kettlebell.

Foundational movements such as the swing, clean and jerk, or snatch are best performed over a period of time. Try to complete fitness movements such as the overhead press, squat, row or deadlift as a set of the repetitions.

An effective way to train for a set period of time is by using the "ladder" protocol.

Example: clean and press for 3 minutes

5 reps on the left side, then 5 reps on the right side
4 reps on the left side, then 4 reps on the right side
3 reps on the left side, then 3 reps on the right side
2 reps on the left side, then 2 reps on the right side
then swing switch back and forth performing 2 reps until 3 minutes has elapsed.

The follow are merely examples. Feel free to contact us for additional suggestions.

Note: Jim Talo can be contacted at www.humanmotion.com.

KETTLEBELL CARDIO ROUTINE

Repeat this series of exercises for 35 to 60 minutes, resting one minute each time you complete an exercise. Decrease the rest period to 30 seconds as you become more efficient.

1 **1/2 Get-Up:** 5 reps (left/right)   Page 31

2 Walk, jog, jumping jacks for 1 minute

3 **Swings**: two-handed, 15 reps (left/right)   Page 21

4 Walk, jog, jumping jacks for 1 minute

5 **Swings**: one-handed, 15 reps (left/right)   Page 20

6 Walk, jog, jumping jacks for 1 minute

7 **1/2 Get-Up:** 5 reps (left/right)   Page 31

8 Walk, jog, jumping jacks for 1 minute

9 **Overhead Push Press:** 5 reps (left/right)   Page 24

10 **Swings**: one-handed, 15 reps (left/right)   Page 20

11 Walk, jog, jumping jacks for 1 minute

12 **Bent-Over Row:** 5 reps (left/right)   Page 42

13 **Swings**: one-handed, 15 reps (left/right)   Page 20

62

KETTLEBELL ENDURANCE ROUTINE

Repeat this series of exercises for 35 to 60 minutes, resting one minute each time you complete an exercise. Decrease the rest period to 30 seconds as you become more efficient.

1 **Turkish Get-Up:** for 4 minutes
(switch sides each time)
Stop performing before becoming fatigued.
 Page 32

2 **Swing:** two handed for 30 seconds,
then left handed for 30 seconds,
then right for 30 seconds, then
switches for 30 seconds.
Page 21

3 **Clean - Squat - Switch:**
Continue for two minutes.

Page 23
Page 35
Page 22

4 **Swing:** left side for 45 seconds,
then right side for 45 seconds.
Page 20

5 **Clean and Press:**
Use ladder protocol 5,4,3,2
(page 60).
Page 23
Page 24

6 **Bent-Over or Planked Row:**
Use ladder protocol 5,4,3,2
(page 60).
Page 42
Page 44

7 **Clean - Squat - Switch:**
Continue for two minutes.
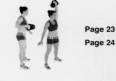
Page 23
Page 35
Page 22

8 **Snatches:**
Continue for two minutes.
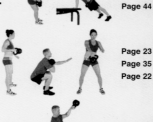
Page 51

KETTLEBELL FITNESS ROUTINE

Note: it is important to practice new techniques before incorporating them in your routine or repeat circuit.

(1) **Split Lunge:** (left/right) Repeat 8-12 reps to muscular fatigue. Page 34

(2) **Double Overhead Press:** Repeat 8-12 reps to muscular fatigue. Page 27

(3) **Face the Wall Squat:** Repeat 8-12 reps to muscular fatigue. Page 37

(4) **Floor Press Double-Arm:** Repeat 8-12 reps to muscular fatigue. Page 30

(5) **Bent-Over Row:** Repeat 8-12 reps to muscular fatigue. Page 42

(6) **Single-Leg Pick Up (left/right):** Repeat 8-12 reps to muscular fatigue. Page 53

(7) **Twisting Crunch (left/right):** Repeat 8-12 reps to muscular fatigue. Page 56

(8) **Bridge with Towel:** Repeat 8-12 reps to muscular fatigue. Page 57

64 Other Products by
Productive Fitness Products Inc.

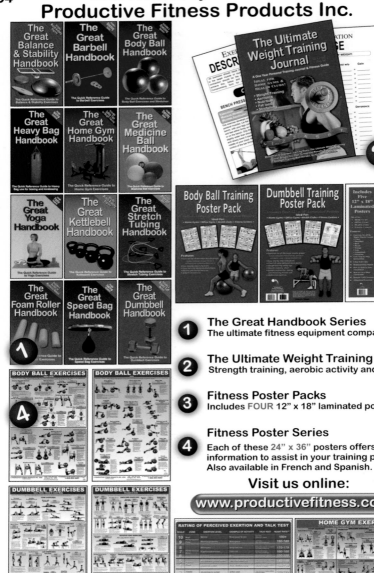
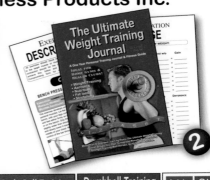
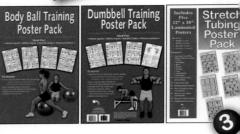

The Great Handbook Series
The ultimate fitness equipment companions.

The Ultimate Weight Training Journal
Strength training, aerobic activity and nutrition

Fitness Poster Packs
Includes FOUR 12" x 18" laminated posters.

Fitness Poster Series
Each of these 24" x 36" posters offers specialized information to assist in your training program. Also available in French and Spanish.

Visit us online:

www.productivefitness.com

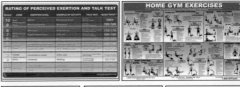
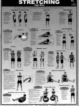
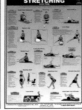
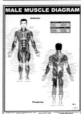
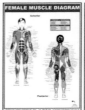
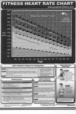